The Hair Edges Manual

A Step By Step Guide For Growing Back The Edges Of Your Hair

AUTHOR BREANNA RUTTER

TABLE OF CONTENTS

INTRODUCTION TO
THE HAIR EDGES MANUAL

"The Hair Edges Manual is a pocket guide that will help you to successfully grow back the edges of your hair. There are a variety of reasons that could have caused you to lose the edges of your hair such as; health issues, aggressive styling, or a natural progression of thinning. Growing back the edges of your hair is a process that can include a wide array of solutions that range from topical edge treatments, a diet high in certain vitamins and nutrients, or the option to go the surgical route! Understanding how to grow back the edges of your hair can be quite challenging especially when patience comes into play because it is required to wait a period of time in conjunction with the natural growth cycle of your hair.

This manual breaks down growing back the edges of your hair in simple easy steps involving growth treatments, hair care regimens and foods that lead to growth and much more! The skills required to growing back the edges of your hair are of a minimum skill level paired with a vast array of hair knowledge so that you can understand why you have to do certain things to your hair, to maintain and encourage the health of it. This manual is here to thoroughly educate you about your hair edges as well as provide a multitude of solutions that will help you to grow back your hair.

Please enjoy this informative read and remain patient throughout the process as you are growing back the edges of your hair!"

Sincerely Breanna

1 HAIR GROWTH CYCLE

Understanding the life cycle of hair will give you the basic foundation of knowing how to diagnose a variety of problems you may encounter when growing healthy hair and achieving your goal lengths. Knowing the behavioral characteristics of hair growth will indicate whether or not your hair is growing, if the shedding you are experiencing is normal and also how quickly you can expect to see growth results. Knowing how long you should expect your edges to grow in is crucial towards knowing if your growing efforts are really making difference!

Hair encounters three stages within its growth or life cycle. Each individual hair you are growing on your head can be in different stages of its life cycle and because of that, you lose on average 80 to 100 strands of hair daily. Given that you have about 100,000 strands of hair on your head in total, don't be alarmed about shedding that many strands because this is a normal process that has to take place. If you think about it, shedding makes up way less than 1% of hair that you have on your scalp right now! Now let's discuss the life cycle of hair.

The Anagen Phase is the 1st phase of the hair life cycle as this is the growing phase because a new hair has begun growing. Since all of your hair is not in the Anagen Phase at once, it will take time before you will notice thickness because other hairs have to enter this phase as well. This phase lasts 2 to 6 years.

The Catagen Phase is the 2nd phase in which your hair is transitioning towards the Telogen phase. The hair is separating from your follicle (see definition guide) and moving upward towards your pore, or the surface of your scalp to fall out as shed hair. This phase lasts 1 to 2 weeks.

The Telogen Phase is the 3rd phase in which the hair is resting because the dermal papilla (see definition guide) separates from the follicle and then moves upward to begin growing a brand new hair. This phase lasts 2 to 4 months.

It is important that you completely understand the hair growth cycle so that you can gauge how long it should take for the edges of your hair to begin showing growth! The Telogen Phase and the Anagen Phase are the only two phases that allows you to see growth in hair. The time frames between the two phases are 2 months to 6 years. You should not have to wait 6 years to see your edges grow because remember, all hair is not in the same phase at the same time!

The golden time frame to stick with when trying different things to growing back the edges of your hair is no longer than 2 to 4 months time to notice growth. You should see growth in as little as 2 months and if you do not see growth, 4 months is the longest time you need to wait to see results of growth.

If you have remained consistent in trying a specific recommendation as instructed for growing your edges, and you see no signs of growth within 2 to 4 months, go ahead and try another recommendation until you find success with growing back the edges of your hair!

2 UNDERSTANDING HAIR PH

Have you experienced difficulty maintaining smooth frizz free hair? Frizzy hair will ruin any hairstyle and the common situations that cause frizzy poofy hair is when straight, in braids, or in twists. The reason why frizzy hair is hard to beat is because the hair is not PH balanced! PH balance has a lot to do with the health and behavior of your hair to achieve certain results. In relation to the edges of your hair, your hair is left prone to breakage if it is not in its ideal range of PH!

The PH scale is used to measure how acidic or alkaline a solution is and the scale ranges from 1 (acidic) to 14 (alkaline). Water has a PH of 7 (neutral) and is used to compare the acidity or alkalinity of a solution. The ideal PH range of hair is 4.5 to 5.5. Hair has an acidity of 4.5 to 5.5 and should remain this way especially if you want to achieve your most healthy hair. The reason why this is important is because when your hair is in contact with an acidic product, it will cause your cuticles (refer to definition guide) to flatten resulting in smooth & healthy moisturized strands of hair. When hair is in contact with an alkaline solution, the cuticles raise, the strands themselves swell (which can cause breakage) resulting in rough & frizzy dry hair.

When caring for your hair edges, it is high priority to always keep your hair in the range of 4.5 to 5.5 and a great way to do this, is to make sure that your hair care products are PH balanced. If you do not know the PH of your hair care products, test your products with Litmus Strips. You can find these strips in specialty stores and online. If you want products that are already PH balanced, I highly suggest HowToBlackHair.com referred hair care products specifically formulated for maintaining healthy hair.

3 EDGES HAIR GROWTH OILS

There are a multitude of hair care products available on the market that offer to repair a variety of hair problems many individuals suffer from today. Visit a local drug store to check out the beauty isle to inspect the hair care products. You will notice that most of the hair care products offer repair for problems such as split ends, fading color, flat thin hair and so on! The problem is that many products that promise hair growth are not actually formulated with ingredients that contribute to the growth of your hair. When reading the labels of many commercialized hair care products, you will notice that the most popular products are filled with ingredients such as; petrolatum, silicones, and sulfates! These are the worst ingredients known for hair because they cause buildup, breakage, and dry hair! To grow back the edges of your hair, it is best to make sure that you are using ingredients that strengthen your hair from the inside out, encourage blood flow for optimal hair growth, and keep your hair PH balanced.

On the following pages are recipes for edges hair growth oils and a regimen that you can use and follow along with in the comfort of your own home to help you grow back the edges of your hair. Please keep in mind the growth cycle of hair is in between 2 months to 6 years so give yourself 2 to 4 months, courtesy of the Anagen Phase, to truly see results of hair growth. If one recipe does not improve your hair as suggested, move onto another edge treatment after 4 months to find the solution that works for you!

Always perform a 24 hour patch test in a discrete area of your head. All recipes contribute to hair growth but some also offer the benefit of treating other hair problem as well!

EDGES HAIR OIL RECIPES
(always 24 hour patch test for sensitivity)

Thoroughly mix any given solution in its own applicator bottle and store spout covered with its cap to prevent the evaporation of essential oil!

Rosemary Recipe
(For Growth)

- 5 drops Rosemary Essential Oil
- 1 oz/2 tbsp Virgin Cold Pressed Coconut Oil

Ylang Ylang Recipe
(For Strength)

- 5 drops Ylang Ylang Essential Oil
- 1 oz/2 tbsp Organic Sesame Oil

Peppermint Recipe
(For Increased Blood Flow)

- 5 drops Peppermint Essential Oil
- 1 oz/2 tbsp Organic Safflower Oil

Lavender Recipe
(For Inflammation)

- 5 drops Lavender Essential Oil
- 1 oz/2 tbsp Virgin Cold Pressed Olive Oil

Tea Tree Recipe
(For Dandruff/Itchiness)

- 5 drops Tea Tree Essential Oil
- 1 oz/2 tbsp Virgin Cold Pressed Grapeseed Oil

Jamaican Recipe
(For Growth + Strength)

- 1 oz/2 tbsp Organic Jamaican Black Castor Oil

EDGES HAIR OIL APPLICATION + REGIMEN

THIS CAN BE DONE DAILY!

Step #1 Moisten edges with a water spray bottle, wait a couple of minutes and GENTLY separate edges from the rest of your hair with your fingers. If applicable, apply the same instructions to your nape hair as well

Step #2 Lubricate your fingers with your Edges Hair Oil Recipe of choice and GENTLY smooth onto your edges

Allow some of the treatment to base your scalp as well for stimulation!

Step #3 If possible, GENTLY two strand twist a 1/2 inch to 1 inch sections of edges to avoid additional manipulation from styling

If not possible, leave hair as is

DO NOT STYLE YOUR EDGES OR APPLY ADDITIONAL PRODUCT WHATSOEVER!

4 DETANGLE REGIMEN

The Detangling Regimen for the edges of your hair is a vital technique that must be done appropriately every single time you need to detangle your hair! Detangling your hair should never be performed often and improperly for a couple of reasons; excessive detangling causes breakage and constant detangling overtime leads to thinning. The most difficult part about detangling has always been encountering knots and tangles and even more daunting than that, grooming thick or course hair!

Thick Hair: your ponytail width, with all of your hair gathered, is the width of a quarter or larger

Course Hair: your individual strands of hair are the same size or bigger in size (diameter) to regular sewing thread

Even if you do not have thick and/or course hair, that does not mean detangling fine or thin hair is any easier. When it comes to hair of this kind, minimum breakage and tangles look very pronounced and even more difficult to conceal!

Thin Hair: your ponytail width, with all of your hair gathered, is the width of a nickel or smaller

Fine Hair: your individual strands of hair are smaller in size (diameter) to regular sewing thread

Provided next is a detangling regimen for the edges of your hair whether or not you have much of any edges or not. For more, check out the The Transitioning Hair Manual, The Relaxed Hair Bible, or The Natural Hair Bible if you need detailed hair care instructions and hair care regimens for growing longer and healthier hair.

DETANGLE REGIMEN FOR HAIR EDGES

Step #1 Moisten edges with a water spray bottle, wait a couple of minutes and GENTLY separate edges from the rest of your hair with your fingers. If applicable, apply the same instructions to your nape hair as well

Step #2 If possible, GENTLY two strand twist a 1/2 inch to 1 inch section of edges. If not possible, leave any edge hair smoothed forward

Step #3 Detangle the rest of your hair if you need to perform your Hair Care Regimen (refer to the appropriate hair care bible)

Step #4 Perform your Hair Care Regimen to your hair edges without detangling or unraveling your edges

Step #5 Finish by lubricating your edges and scalp with you Edge Hair Oil of choice

DO NOT STYLE YOUR EDGES OR APPLY
ADDITIONAL PRODUCT WHATSOEVER!

5 NIGHT TIME ROUTINE

Your night time routine is vital for preserving the health of your hair and without this routine, you will constantly suffer from breakage. Not only does handling your hair in a gentle manner dramatically decrease breakage, but so does your protective night time routine!

When performing your night time routine, it is very important that the edges of your hair have been already prepped with your Edge Hair Oil Application. Before going to bed, you must always protect with appropriate material to eliminate friction encountered throughout the night. The two choices of fabric that are best for protecting your hair throughout the night are Satin and Silk.

Satin is more affordable than silk, is the more flexible material and can be washed with ease. Satin does not cause friction on your hair or edges and nor does Silk, but Satin causes more friction in comparison to Silk.

Silk is priced higher than satin, is not as flexible in comparison and has to be delicately hand washed or cleansed through a dry cleaning service. Silk does not cause friction on your hair or edges and nor does Satin, but Silk is superior in preventing friction than Satin.

There are a few ways to protect your hair from friction with Silk or Satin material such as using a; Satin/Silk Pillowcase, Bonnet or Head Scarf. For growing back the edges of your hair, it is preferred to sleep with a Bonnet or Scarf to keep the hair neat with no movement throughout the night.

Following the suggested regimen allows you to protect the edges of your hair to eliminate friction and breakage.

NIGHT TIME ROUTINE

Step #1 Perform The Edges Hair Oil Application

Step #2 (For Satin/Silk Pillowcase)

Cover your bed pillow of choice with your case of choice. Double case your pillow if needed because of slippage.

Step #3 (For Satin/Silk Bonnet)

Wear a comfortable but secure bonnet that covers all of the edges of your hair If the bonnet feels tight or too loose to stay secure, seek another bonnet or protection of choice.

Step #4 (For Satin/Silk Head Scarf)

Secure your scarf around your head in a way that covers all of your hair including your edges.

IMPORTANT Alternate the tied knot of your head scarf in a new position on your hairline every night. Constantly knotting the scarf at the same point along your hairline can lead to thinning!

6 HAIRSTYLING OPTIONS

You must carefully consider your choice of extensions and how much manipulation is required to complete a look you desire as well as preserve the health of your gentle edges. Often times, hairstyling is the culprit to many who lost the edges of their hair! Below are lists of some of the worst and best hairstyles to wear to help you grow back the edges of your hair. One important thing to remember is that the more hairs contained within a given braid or twist, the stronger your hair will be in numbers.

WORST HAIRSTYLES FOR THIN EDGES
Micro Braids – small braids cause breakage easily
Kinky Twist (small) – small twists cause breakage easily
Ponytail Sew In – exposed hair edges/nape can break easily
Partial Sew In – leave out experiences breakage easily
Yarn Braids – yarn is too heavy for unhealthy edges
Yarn Wraps – yarn is too heavy for unhealthy edges
U-Part/L-Part Wig – leave out experiences breakage easily
Quick Weave – unhealthy edges will tear from glue removal

THE BEST HAIRSTYLES FOR THIN EDGES
Jumbo Individual Braids – large braids decrease breakage
Kinky Twists (large) – large twists decrease breakage
Net Weave Full Sew In – tension is on net instead of edges
Invisible Part Sew In – smooth edges instead when finished

Even though there are more choices than listed here for best hairstyles, it is most important to leave edges as is without additional hair products or tensions from weaves, extensions, braids or twists. Opt to slick down the edges of your hair while damp with a molding strip instead of applying tension from styles. It will not hold as well as using hair gel but you can use hair gel once you gain healthy edges.

7 HEAT USAGE

Using heat on the edges of your hair is dangerous towards preserving the health of your hairs! Heat should only be used rarely even on healthy hair so when it comes to growing healthy edges, using heat is never appropriate for the most part. The only time heat usage is appropriate is if you are doing a Deep Conditioning or Protein Treatment. In this case, heat is used all over you hair to encourage your products to penetrate your hair. If the heat is focused on the edges of your hair, this will cause your hair to become weakened which results in thinning or breakage.

Some individuals think that if you use heat regularly with a heat protectant it will prevent any cause of breakage when this is totally false! First, before you even bring yourself to using a heat straightener or heat styling tool on your hair, you have to test which setting is best for you. Your preferred heat setting of choice should be the lowest setting on your styling tool that allows you to achieve your straightest result. For some, especially with fine or thin hair, their heat setting usually falls somewhere between 300° and 320° degrees. For those usually with thick or coarse hair, their heat setting will usually fall between 320° to 350°

On healthy hair, moderating your frequency of heat usage, along with using a heat protectant product at your lowest straightening heat setting that works for you, should protect your hair from heat damage. The only way the above suggestion will damage your hair is if your hair is unhealthy! Unhealthy hair is on the brink of breakage and that is why if you want to grow your edges back, you have to stay away from anything and everything that can sacrifice any progress you are trying to make in regards to the health of your hair.

8 CHEMICAL RELAXERS

Some of those who are reading this manual may have relaxed hair and relaxing your hair should not ruin your edges if done appropriately. Always use chemical relaxers with caution and stretch your touch ups as far apart from one another as possible because breakage is always a risk when chemically relaxing your hair.

Chemical relaxers and their dangers are heavily discussed in my book, The Relaxed Hair Bible: The 10 Commandments of Long Healthy Relaxed Hair so if you want to learn concentrated information on their usage, regimens, hair care treatments and more, refer to that book for detailed information. It's important to understand the dangers of using chemical relaxers when trying to grow the edges of your hair. Since this manual is focused on growing your edges and doing everything possible to grow them back healthy, it is suggested to stop chemically relaxing your hair!

This may be hard advice to follow for those who chose to chemically relax their hair. If you choose to postpone your touch ups until you have attained healthy edges you will guarantee yourself the most success with your hair growth. As discussed in the Relaxed Hair Bible, chemical relaxers are highly alkaline and by nature, they disintegrate (or break down) your hairs to the point of straightness. When a relaxer is left on for too long or too high of strength is used, this can cause your hair to melt or simply break off. As mentioned in chapter two titled, Understanding Hair PH, hair is best healthy when kept in the PH range of 4.5 to 5.5 and relaxers have a PH range of 11-14! This is highly corrosive but is used to cause permanent "controlled damage" to your hair and because of this, you should wait until your edges become healthy before relaxing again.

9 EATING FOR HAIR GROWTH

Eating for hair growth is a natural byproduct of eating a diet high in nutrients, minerals, and vitamins! Dieting for hair growth encourages better eating habits that can make you a healthier individual for a lifetime. A diet only lasts as long as you are willing to accept restrictions so opt instead for food choices that you can stick with for life and actually enjoy. The problem with dieting or only eating specific foods for hair growth it that it puts you in a position to ignore foods that you actually enjoy, even if they aren't the healthiest! The key to eating for hair growth is to constantly rotate your favorite foods of choice and more importantly, flavor them in different ways that allows for you to taste as though you are eating something uniquely different.

Before altering your food choices or planning a new eating lifestyle, it's important to know what foods contain the vitamins, minerals and nutrients responsible for actually growing your hair. On the previous page are a list of vitamins and nutrients provided for you along with information on what it does for your hair as well as a list of food suggestions that contain high amounts of these ingredients. Refer to the Dieting For Hair Growth Manual for detailed instructions and information on creating a hair growth diet unique to your hair growth and caloric needs!

VITAMINS & NUTRIENTS
FOR HAIR GROWTH

Omega 3 Fatty Acid – improves scalp blood circulation
Omega 6 Fatty Acid – controls eczema and scalp conditions
Omega 9 Fatty Acid – increases hair elasticity
Vitamin B12 – oxygenates blood vessels of hair shaft base
Vitamin B7 (Biotin or Vitamin H) – reverses hair loss
Vitamin B6 – stops DHT production which thins hair

FOODS HIGH IN HAIR GROWTH
VITAMINS AND NUTRIENTS

OMEGA 3	OMEGA 6	OMEGA 9
Flax Seeds 133%	Brazil Nuts 377%	Safflower Oil 77%
Walnuts 113%	Sunflower Seeds 473%	Olive Oil 75%
Sardines 61%	Pine Nuts 32%	Peanut Oil 48%
Flaxseed Oil 57%		

VITAMIN B12	VITAMIN B7	VITAMIN B6
Clams 1041%	Peanuts 88%	Sunflower Seeds 94%
Beef Liver 1178%	Almonds 49%	Salmon 40%
Bran Cereal 300%	Sweet Potato 29%	Banana 41%
Mackerel 269%	Egg Yolk 27%	

% = percentage of nutritional value per serving based on
the requirements of a 2,000 calorie diet

Eating healthy not only strengthens your body inwardly, but excess vitamins and nutrients are delivered to your skin, nails, and hair! Have you ever heard about or seen the "glow" of a pregnant woman? Women who are pregnant experience healthier skin, nails and hair and this is due part to an increase in vitamins, nutrients and minerals from their prenatal pills. Non-pregnant women are not suggested to take prenatals because the high levels of iron can cause many to feel constipated so it's better to take a multi vitamin instead. Taking a multi vitamin or adult vitamin allows for your body to absorb vitamins, nutrients and minerals that you may have missed through your diet. The best way to get in all of your vitamins, minerals and nutrients is to research what a healthy diet is for a woman (or man) of your age, height and BMI (Body Mass Index).

Multi vitamins and a more popular supplement called Biotin (also called Vitamin H or B7), will contribute greatly to the growth of your hair. Biotin unlike multi vitamins, are a blend of various B vitamins that contribute most to the growth of your hair. In contrast, adult vitamins are a blend of all the necessary vitamins, nutrients, and minerals that your body needs to remain healthy. Compare them to healthy foods for example, Biotin can represent peanuts for example (since peanuts are high in Vitamin B7) and Adult vitamins can represent a balanced diet (fruits, vegetables, meats and carbohydrates). Having a balanced diet, or wide array of vitamins, allows for you to reap more health benefits in general than consuming just a blend of B Vitamins.

If you want to eat specifically for hair growth, check out the Dieting For Hair Growth Manual for detailed instructions and information on creating a hair growth diet plan.

10 THINNING WITH AGE

Many of us wish that we could never age or feel the weight of aging on our bodies and minds but unfortunately, we will all age with every passing year. When you are young and energetic, your body has the ability to handle infections, viruses, diseases and injuries phenomenally better than your body can in old age. The benefit also to being younger is a higher metabolism that helps to maintain a more fit body, tighter more youthful skin, and a head full of hair!

Many women and men who age notice that their hair becomes thinner as time passes and this is most noticeable to those who remembered having a thick head full of hair in their younger days. The reason why many of an older age begin to have thinning hair is because your hormonal balance changes within your body. As you age, your hormones aren't raging as much as they used to in young age and because of this, estrogen levels will begin to decrease after a certain age , usually starting in your late 20's to mid 30's. As estrogen levels within the body decrease overtime, in both men and women, this leads to a production of DHT. As you age, its effects are what we visually see as pattern baldness.

DHT (Dihydrotestosterone): an enzyme that develops with the conversion of testosterone and Type II 5-alpha reductase, which is located in the oil gland of your hair follicle

Pattern baldness is a normal encounter many will or can endure with their hair and if this is not the reason for your loss of edges, but you still want to learn how to revert this problem, refer to the How To Fix Thinning Hair Manual.

11 SURGICAL HAIR RESTORATION

Surgical hair restoration is only suggested for those who have truly given every home made remedy and diet plan a fair and independent chance. Before going under the knife, give each individual Edge Hair Oil Recipe and a diet rich in specific vitamins and nutrients its chance to produce results within a time frame of 2 to 4 months.

Taking a natural approach to growing back the edges of your hair is at a lower price point than surgery can offer but it is still completely up to you and understandable to seek surgical hair restoration. There are two options you can take to surgically restore your edge hairs permanently!

FUE Hair Transplant: Follicular Unit Extraction
FUT Hair Transplant: Follicular Unit Transplant

The FUE transplant requires individual follicles to be extracted from your scalp after injecting a local anesthesia to the preferred area of extraction. This procedure involves implanting individual follicles throughout your thinning or bald area of scalp. The positives to this procedure is that it does not require staples/stiches, leaves behind no scars, and requires little recovery time. The negative is that it can take multiple procedures to achieve your desired result of density.

The FUT transplant requires a thin patch of scalp removed preferably from the back of your head after injecting a local anesthesia. This procedure involves dissecting your scalp into patches of 2 to 4 follicle units that will be inserted into your desired scalp area. The positive of this procedure is that it can be done in one session. The negative is that it can leave behind a scar, requires staples/stiches and has a lengthy recovery time.

AFTERWORDS

"This manual was made in mind for those who desire step by step help with growing back the edges of their hair in a way that allows you to try a variety of solutions. As you may have read throughout these chapters, this manual is condensed with a wide variety of solutions for achieving healthy edge hairs that you may seem to lack. You may have chosen to read this guide because you support my work, you were looking for information on growing your edges, or you were looking for this information to help a loved one.

Personally, I have never had problems with the edges of my hair but what is to be noted is that the edges of my hair and the nape are a little bit finer and at a lower density than the rest of my hair. This does not bother me and I have never had problems with breakage or thinning on my edges because I take great care of my hair and something that has been golden for retaining length on my edges hairs, has been from two strand twisting medium to small sections of just my edge hairs. I constantly receive an overwhelming amount of emails daily from women and men, who need help with their hair and the majority of these emails, consist of help with growing back the edges of their hair. This manual is inspired by those who need my help in this way.

I hope that you thoroughly enjoyed this read, it was a pleasure of mine to write this for your knowledge and enjoyment."

Sincerely, Breanna

ADDITIONAL RESOURCES

The Official Website: www.Howtoblackhair.com

The Online Store: www.HowtoblackhairStore.com

Free Subscription Email: http://eepurl.com/FZs5b

For Additional Hair Questions

YourHairQuestions@Gmail.com

Black Hair Styling Tutorials

BlackWomenHair YouTube Channel

www.Youtube.com/BlackWomenHair

HowToBlackHair YouTube Channel

www.Youtube.com/HowToBlackHair

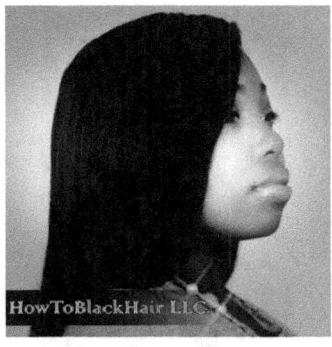

The Natural Hair Bible

The 10 Commandments of Black Hair Care

www.HowToBlackHair.com

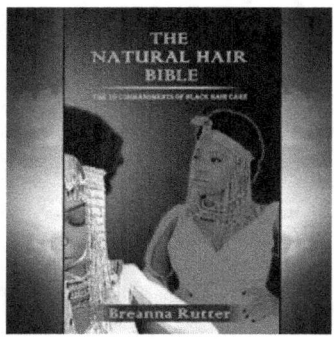

The Relaxed Hair Bible

The 10 Commandments of Long Healthy Relaxed Hair

www.HowToBlackHair.com

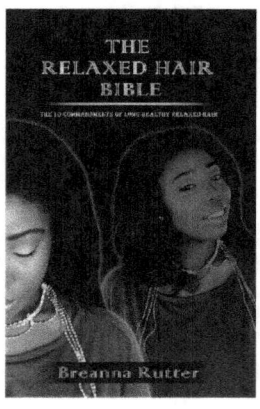

Black Hair Styling DVDs (Over 20+ Hairstyles)

www.HowToBlackHair.com

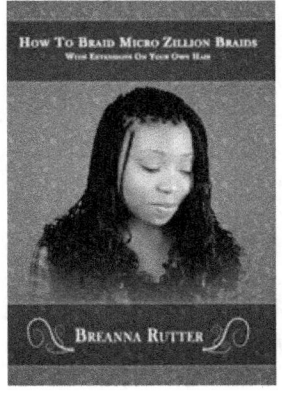 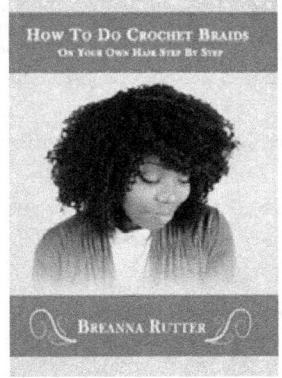

DEFINITION GUIDE

Anagen: *the growth phase of the hair cycle*

Catagen: *the transitioning phase of the hair cycle*

Course Hair: your individual strands of hair are the same size or bigger in size (diameter) to regular sewing thread

Cuticles: *a naturally protecting shield (arranged like shingles to the roof of a home) outside of your hair strands*

Dermal Papilla: *a raised dermis located underneath the root of your follicle that houses the blood supply*

DHT (Dihydrotestosterone): *an enzyme that becomes from the conversion of testosterone and Type II 5-alpha reductase located in the oil gland of your hair follicle*

Follicle: *an individual strand of hair*

Fine Hair: *your individual strands of hair are smaller in size (diameter) to regular sewing thread*

FUE Hair Transplant: *Follicular Unit Extraction*

FUT Hair Transplant: *Follicular Unit Transplant*

Hair Life Cycle: *the cycle of hair growth*

PH Balance: *hair balanced with a PH of 4.5 to 5.5*

Shedding: *natural hair loss experienced from the catagen to telogen phase*

Telogen: *the rest phase of the hair cycle*

Thick Hair: *your ponytail width, with all of your hair gathered, is the width of a quarter or larger*

Thin Hair: *your ponytail width, with all of your hair gathered, is the width of a nickel or smaller*

INDEX

TESTOSTERONE: *22 & 28*
VITAMINS: *23*

HOW TO BLACK HAIR LLC.
WRITTEN BY BREANNA RUTTER
BOOK DESIGNED BY BREANNA RUTTER
COVER DESIGNED BY JARED RUTTER
ALL RIGHTS RESERVED.
VISIT WWW.HOWTOBLACKHAIR.COM

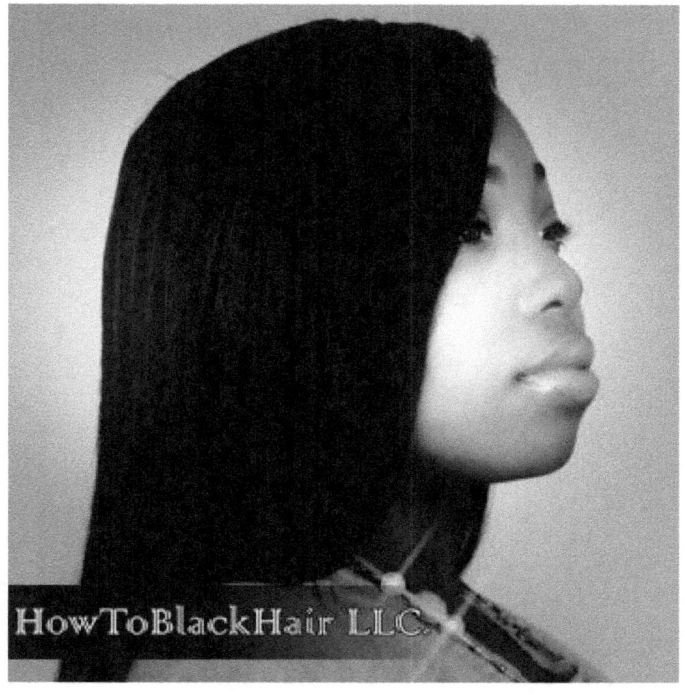